KOY KUT

Hair on The Mind

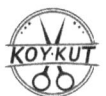

Copyright © 2025 by Koy Kut

All rights reserved. No part of this publication may be reproduced, stored or transmitted in any form or by any means, electronic, mechanical, photocopying, recording, scanning, or otherwise without written permission from the publisher. It is illegal to copy this book, post it to a website, or distribute it by any other means without permission.

First edition

This book was professionally typeset on Reedsy. Find out more at reedsy.com

For everyone who ever looked in the mirror and doubted themselves.
For those who learned to love their reflection anyway.
This book is for you.

"What's on your head reflects what's on your mind"

                                          Koy Kut

Contents

Foreword — iii
Preface — iv
Acknowledgments — v
Prologue — 1
Introduction — 2

I Roots & Identity

1. Roots Run Deep — 7
2. The First Cut Hurt — 9
3. Hair as Identity — 12
4. The Pressure to Fit In — 15

II Hair, Healing & Mental Health

5. The Big Chop — 19
6. Growth Takes Time — 21
7. Stress, Trauma & Hair Loss — 24
8. The Mirror Test — 27

III Myths & Empowerment

9. Hair & Social Media Pressure — 33
10. The CROWN Act — 35

11	Barbershop & Salon Therapy	37
12	The Gender Hair Divide	40
13	Hair & Relationships	42
14	Hair & Aging	45
15	Money, Hair & Hustle	47
16	Hair as Celebration	49

IV	Society, Culture & Connection	
17	Myths We Grew Up On	55
18	Slay The Day, The Hair Way	58

Epilogue	61
About the Author	64

Foreword

Hair is never just hair. It carries history, identity, pride, and sometimes pain. It's the first thing people notice about us, and often the first thing we notice about ourselves. A cut can change our whole mood. A style can shift our confidence. And for so many of us, what we do with our hair says more than words ever could.

This book is about those stories — the ones we've lived, laughed about, or even cried through. It's about the connection between what's on our heads and what's on our minds. Because the truth is, hair and mental health are linked in ways most people don't talk about, but everyone feels.

As you read, you'll see yourself in these pages. You'll remember the first cut that made you feel unstoppable, and the one that made you want to hide under a hat. You'll think about the pressure to fit in, and the freedom that comes when you stop asking for permission to be yourself.

What you hold in your hands is more than a book. It's a mirror. One that reflects not just styles and trends, but growth, healing, and confidence.

Because hair grows. Styles fade. But self-love? That lasts forever.

Preface

I didn't write this book to tell you how to style your hair. I wrote it because I've seen, over and over again, how much hair connects to who we are and how we feel. As a barber, I've watched people walk into the chair carrying stress, doubt, and insecurity — and walk out lighter, smiling, confident again. And I've learned that what happens in the mirror is about more than just a cut.

This book is about those moments. The times a style gave you courage. The times a bad cut made you want to hide. The pressure to fit in, and the freedom of finally being yourself. Hair is a thread that runs through all of it — identity, culture, confidence, and mental health.

I want you to read these chapters like conversations. Like sitting in the chair and sharing stories, laughing, reflecting, maybe even healing a little. Some chapters will feel like your own life. Others might open your eyes to experiences you never thought about. But all of them are meant to remind you of one thing: you are more than what's on your head.

Hair grows. Styles change. But how you carry yourself — that's what lasts.

— Koy Kut

Acknowledgments

This book wasn't written alone. Every client who's ever sat in my chair, every story I've heard in the barbershop or salon, every laugh, every vent, every quiet moment of reflection — you're all part of this. Thank you for reminding me that hair is never just hair, it's life, it's therapy, it's confidence.

To my family and friends — thank you for holding me down, encouraging me, and reminding me of my own worth when I needed it most.

To the culture — from braids on the porch to barbershop Saturdays, from twists to fades to locs — thank you for giving us roots deeper than style.

And most importantly, to the reader — thank you for picking this up, for giving these words your time, and for trusting me with a piece of your journey. This book is ours now.

Prologue

The chair squeaks as you sit down. Clippers buzz low in the background, conversations ripple through the shop, and the mirror in front of you waits — ready to show the truth. It's more than a haircut. It's more than a style. In this moment, it feels like the mirror is about to decide who you'll be when you walk out.

We've all been there. Hoping the cut comes out right. Praying the style matches the picture in your head. Because deep down, we know — it's never just hair. It's how we feel about ourselves. It's how the world sees us. It's the difference between walking with your head down and walking with your chest out.

That's where this story begins. Not with products or routines. Not with perfect styles or picture-ready hair. But with the truth: every braid, every twist, every fade, every chop carries weight. And every strand has a story worth telling.

This book is about those stories — the ones we've lived, the ones we've shared in chairs, on porches, in bathrooms, and in mirrors. Stories that remind us that hair grows, styles change, but confidence is what lasts.

And if you're ready to see yourself in a new way, it starts here — in the chair, with the mirror waiting.

Introduction

INTRODUCTION

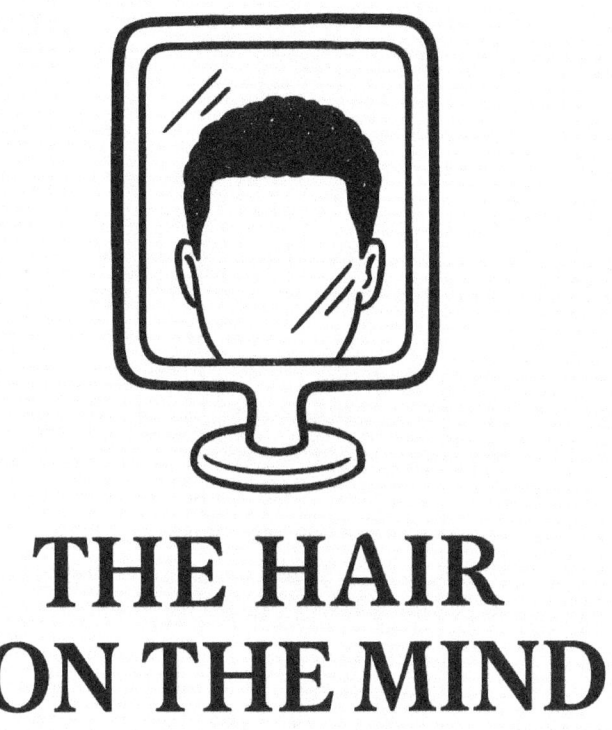

THE HAIR ON THE MIND

*It's never just hair —
it's how you carry yourself.*

You ever stand in the mirror and realize you're not just looking at hair — you're looking at *you*? Not just the cut, not just the curls, but the whole vibe. Some mornings, your hair is undefeated, like it woke up ready to take on the world with you. Other mornings, it's like your hair is in a bad mood — edges won't stay down, curls won't curl, fade won't sit right. We laugh about it, but honestly, those little mirror moments can decide what kind of day we're about to have.

That's because hair has always been more than hair. It's how we introduce ourselves without saying a word. It's culture, it's family, it's identity, and sometimes, it's pressure. From braids done on the porch to that one time somebody told you your style wasn't "professional," hair has always carried more weight than just style.

When your hair is on point, you walk different. Your confidence goes up, you feel untouchable. But when it's off, it's like it follows you everywhere. Truth is, what's on your head often reflects what's on your mind. That's why the way we think about our hair connects so closely to our mental health.

So as you flip these pages, don't expect a "how-to" or some boring lecture. Expect stories. Real ones. Some funny, some deep, all true in their own way. Stories that show how every cut, every braid, every twist carries meaning. And maybe, you'll see a piece of yourself in here — and walk away with a little more love for the head and the hair you carry.

"It's never just hair — it's how you carry yourself."

I

Roots & Identity

1

Roots Run Deep

Think back to your earliest memory of getting your hair done. Maybe it was sitting on the floor between your mom's or grandma's knees, watching cartoons while your scalp got pulled in every direction. Maybe it was that first trip to the barbershop, nervous in the chair, wondering if the cut would come out fresh or have you hiding under a hat.

Those moments felt small back then, but they stick with you. Because hair is one of the first ways we learn about who we are. For some of us, it was culture passed down — braids, twists, locs, cornrows. For others, it was that weekly Saturday cut that made you feel sharp walking into school on Monday. Whatever the story, our "roots" weren't just about hair. They were about identity.

And the messages we got early on? They shaped the way we see ourselves. Maybe you were praised for your hair being "good." Maybe you got teased for it being "nappy." Maybe the hot comb came out every holiday because someone decided your natural curls weren't "done." All of that, whether we realized it or not, sank into us. It taught us something about beauty, about acceptance, about what it meant to fit in.

The truth is, roots run deeper than the scalp. They carry history, family, and memory. They're the start of how we connect hair to our self-worth. And as much as we grow and change, those early messages don't just disappear — they live in the way we see the mirror today.

So think about it: what did your roots teach you? Was it pride? Was it pressure? Was it both? Either way, knowing where it started is the first step to understanding where you stand now.

"Strong roots grow strong branches."

2

The First Cut Hurt

You never forget your first bad haircut. Maybe the barber pushed your line back. Maybe the stylist cut off way more than you asked for. Maybe the curls didn't pop the way you imagined, and suddenly you're staring in the mirror like, *"What did they do to me?"*

HAIR ON THE MIND

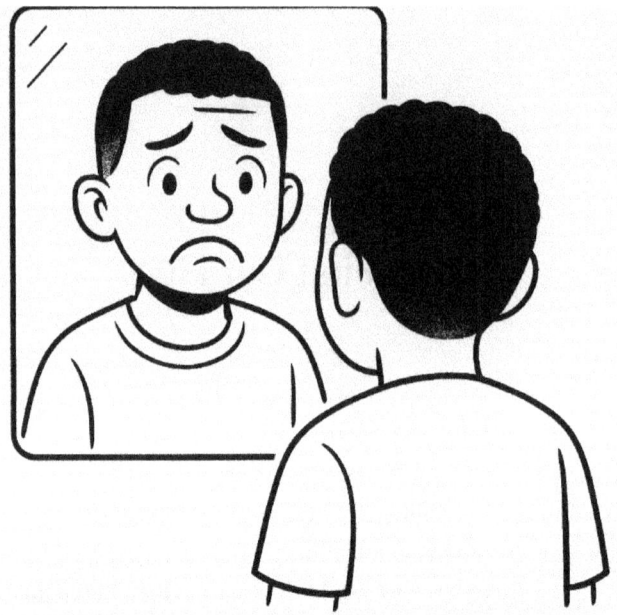

ONE BAD CUT DON'T STOP THE NEXT FADE.

It's wild how something so simple can hit so hard. Because it's not just hair that got cut — it's confidence. That walk back into school or work feels heavier. You feel eyes on you, even if nobody's looking. One slip of the clippers, one wrong snip, and suddenly you're questioning everything.

That's when you realize hair carries power. It decides how we feel in our own skin. It decides if we step out bold or try to hide. And it teaches us something else too: how fragile our self-image can be when it's tied to how we look.

But here's the flip side — the same way a bad cut can break you down, the right one can lift you up. A fresh line, a clean fade, the perfect twist-out — suddenly you feel unstoppable. That's why it matters. Because the mirror doesn't just show us what's on the outside. It reflects how we feel on the inside.

So yeah, the first cut hurts. But it also teaches you resilience. Every "bad hair day" is proof that confidence has to come from deeper than the style. The cut grows back. The style fades. But the way you carry yourself? That's what sticks.

"One bad cut don't stop the next fade."

3

Hair as Identity

Hair has always been more than just style — it's identity. Walk into a room with an Afro, braids, locs, a clean fade, or a silk press, and before you even open your mouth, people already think they know something about you. Sometimes that works in your favor. Sometimes it doesn't.

Maybe you've been praised for rocking your natural look — people telling you how "bold" or "beautiful" it is. Other times, you've been judged, like your style made you "too much" or "not professional." The wild part is, it's the same head of hair, just different eyes looking at it. That's the thing about identity: it's not just how you see yourself, it's how the world reacts to you.

And that's where the pressure kicks in. Hair becomes a silent introduction. A statement without words. A reflection of where you come from and how you want to show up in the world. But here's the catch — if you're not careful, you start living for their approval instead of your own.

HAIR AS IDENTITY

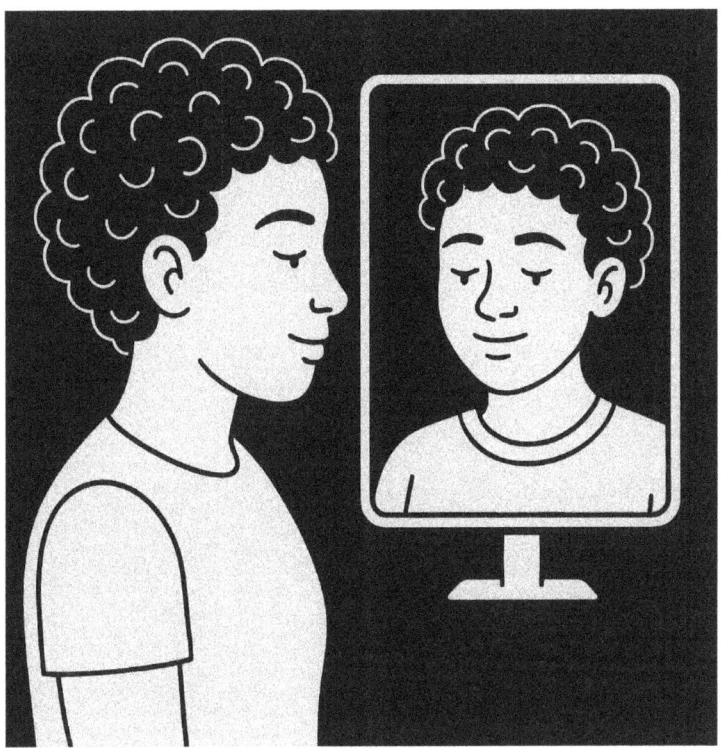

The truth is, your hair can't please everybody. Some will love it. Some will hate it. Some won't understand it at all. But that doesn't change the fact that it's yours. Identity starts when you stop asking for permission and start owning what feels true to you.

So ask yourself: am I wearing this style for me, or for them? If the answer is "for me," then you're already walking in your identity, unapologetically.

"Your hair speaks before you do."

4

The Pressure to Fit In

At some point, almost everybody has felt the pressure to change their hair just to fit in. Maybe it was the straightener heating up on Sunday night before school pictures. Maybe it was the wave cap tied tight because you needed your 360s spinning before the first day back. Maybe it was tucking your curls under a wig or hat because you didn't want the comments.

We don't always admit it, but deep down, we've all wanted to blend in at some point. To not stand out. To not give people another reason to look, to question, to judge. And hair becomes the easiest target. It's right there, on display.

But here's the problem: every time you change yourself for them, a little piece of you disappears. The heat damages more than your curls. The conformity damages your spirit. And the pressure doesn't stop — it just grows heavier the more you give in.

The truth is, trying to meet everyone else's standard is exhausting. It steals your joy, your confidence, your authenticity. And worst of all? It convinces you that who you are naturally isn't enough. That's not fitting in — that's losing yourself.

Fitting in feels safe in the moment. But being yourself lasts longer. Your hair doesn't need their approval. It needs your acceptance.

"Don't burn yourself trying to fit their mold."

II

Hair, Healing & Mental Health

5

The Big Chop

There's a certain silence in the room when the scissors come out and the first chunk of hair hits the floor. Whether it's years of growth or just a style you've been holding onto, the big chop always feels like more than just a haircut. It's a reset.

For some, it happens after heartbreak. For others, it's after damage, stress, or simply being tired of fighting with your hair. Whatever the reason, that first look in the mirror after a big chop hits different. You don't just see less hair — you see yourself stripped down, raw, starting fresh.

And that's the thing: cutting it off is never really about the hair. It's about letting go of what came with it. The weight. The expectations. The old version of you that no longer fits who you're becoming.

It's scary, no doubt. You feel exposed, even vulnerable. But in that vulnerability is power. Power to redefine yourself. Power to say, "This is me now, and I don't need permission to change."

HAIR ON THE MIND

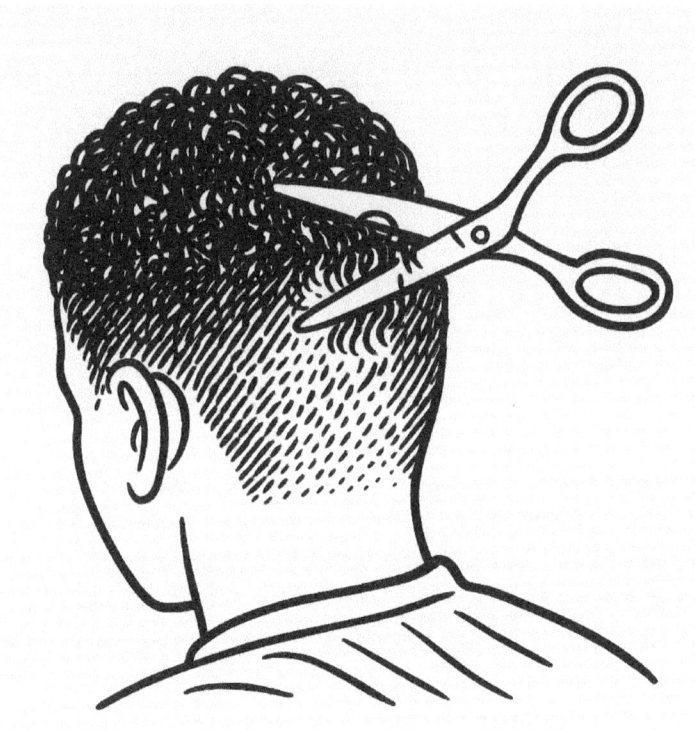

The big chop reminds us that sometimes, to grow, you have to release. The same way dead ends stop your hair from thriving, old baggage stops your spirit from moving forward. When you let go of what's holding you back, you make room for what's waiting to grow.

"Sometimes you gotta cut it off to grow back better."

6

Growth Takes Time

After the chop, the first thing everybody asks is the same: "So how long you think it'll take to grow back?" Like growth can be rushed. Like patience isn't part of the process.

Those first few weeks feel strange. Your hair is shorter, different, maybe even uneven. You check the mirror every morning hoping it stretched overnight, but growth has its own pace. It doesn't care about your timeline. And if you've ever waited on hair to grow, you know it teaches you one thing quick: **Patience.**

YOU'VE GOT TO LET IT GROW

The journey can feel frustrating — watching other people's hair flourish while yours seems stuck, counting inches, trying every oil, every remedy, every trick the internet swears by. But the truth is, no shortcut can change the fact that real growth takes time.

And isn't life the same? Healing after heartbreak, bouncing back from stress, finding yourself again — none of it happens instantly. Just like hair, the roots are working underground before you see results. Progress is quiet before it's visible.

So if you're in that "waiting season," don't lose hope. Growth is happening, even if you can't see it yet. Every inch matters.

GROWTH TAKES TIME

Every small change adds up.

"Good things — and good hair — don't happen overnight."

7

Stress, Trauma & Hair Loss

One of the hardest things to notice is when stress shows up in your hair. At first, it's little — shedding more than usual, edges thinning out, breakage you can't explain. You think it's the products, or maybe the weather. But deep down, it's more than that.

Hair loss has a way of sneaking in during the toughest seasons of life. When you're juggling too much. When the anxiety is nonstop. When grief or heartbreak sits heavy. It's like your body starts telling on you, showing signs of what your mind has been carrying.

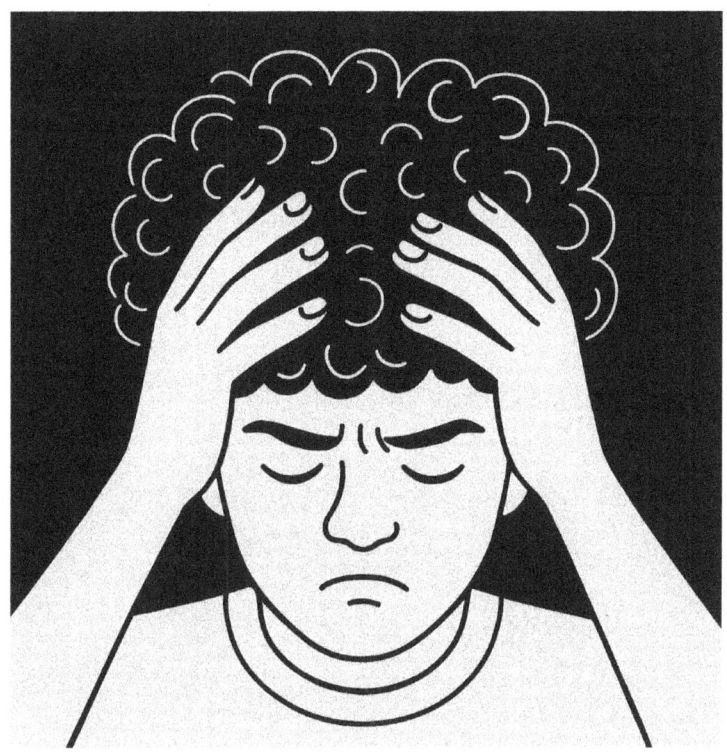

And the thing is, it's not just about looks. It's about identity. Watching your hair fall out or thin can feel like watching your confidence slip away strand by strand. The mirror doesn't just show hair missing — it shows pieces of you that feel missing too.

But here's what's real: hair loss doesn't mean you're broken. It means your body is asking for care. Just like a plant wilts without water, we shrink when we don't tend to know what's going on inside. Healing starts when you stop ignoring the stress and start facing it.

HAIR ON THE MIND

It's not easy, but your worth has never been measured by thickness, edges, or length. You are more than what you see in the mirror. And when your mind heals, your body often follows.

"What's heavy on the mind shows up on the body."

8

The Mirror Test

There's always that moment after a fresh cut or style when you finally face the mirror. The chair spins, the stylist steps back, and it's just you and your reflection. Sometimes you light up instantly — grinning, snapping pics, feeling like the world better be ready. Other times, your face drops. The style isn't what you imagined, or maybe it looks fine but *you* don't feel fine.

HAIR ON THE MIND

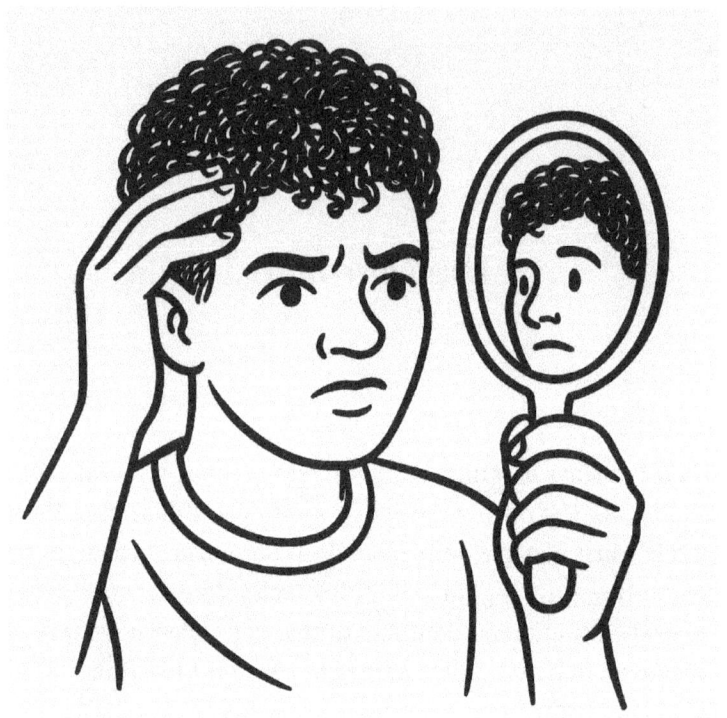

That mirror moment is powerful because it's not just showing hair — it's showing mindset. On the good days, you see confidence. On the rough ones, you see every insecurity. And it's crazy how quick that reflection can change the way you carry yourself for the whole day.

The truth is, the mirror only reflects what your mind projects. If you're already doubting yourself, the mirror will highlight it. If you're standing in self-love, the mirror will magnify it. It's less about the style and more about the story you're telling yourself while you look.

So the next time you face the mirror, pay attention to the

words you say in your head. If they're harsh, flip the script. If they're doubtful, remind yourself who you are beyond the hair. That reflection isn't your enemy — it's your reminder to speak life into yourself.

"The mirror reflects what the mind projects."

III

Myths & Empowerment

9

Hair & Social Media Pressure

Scroll long enough and you'll start to feel it — the pressure. Perfect twist-outs, flawless lace fronts, line-ups so sharp they look airbrushed. Every post looks effortless, but you know behind the scenes it took hours, filters, and maybe even a little Photoshop. Still, you catch yourself comparing.

You start thinking,

"Why don't my curls look like that?" or ***"My fade don't last as long."***

Before you know it, what used to feel normal starts feeling like it's not enough. That's the trap of social media — it magnifies perfection while hiding the reality.

And it's not just about hair. It's about self-worth. When every scroll is a highlight reel, it's easy to forget that real life doesn't look like that 24/7. You're comparing your behind-the-scenes to someone else's best angles, and that's never a fair fight.

The impact runs deep. It's not just hair envy — it's anxiety, it's self-doubt, it's the thought that you need to buy, fix, or hide something just to measure up. But here's the truth: no filter, no likes, no comments can define your beauty. Only you can.

So next time the scroll starts making you question yourself, pause. Remind yourself that your journey is real, even if it's not picture-perfect. Real is always better than curated.

"Don't compare your behind-the-scenes to someone's highlight reel."

10

The CROWN Act

Picture this: you walk into school or work with your hair freshly braided, twisted, or locked, feeling good about yourself. Then someone pulls you aside — maybe a teacher, maybe a boss — and tells you it's "a distraction," "not neat," or "unprofessional." In one moment, what felt normal and beautiful turns into something judged and policed.

This is nothing new. For generations, Black hair has been labeled as a problem in spaces that were never built with us in mind. Straight hair got stamped as "professional." Natural hair, protective styles, and locs got marked as "unacceptable." Respectability politics taught us that to succeed, we had to look less like ourselves and more like somebody else.

That's why movements like the CROWN Act exist — laws that protect people from hair-based discrimination. Because it's not just about style. It's about dignity, identity, and the right to show up as yourself without fear of being punished for it.

But here's the truth: even without the law, wearing your natural hair in spaces that expect you to conform is an act of resistance. Every Afro, every braid, every twist says,

"I am enough as I am."

And that statement is louder than any speech.
    So when the world tries to police your look, remember — they may control the rules, but they don't control your pride.

"They can police the rules, but they can't police your pride."

11

Barbershop & Salon Therapy

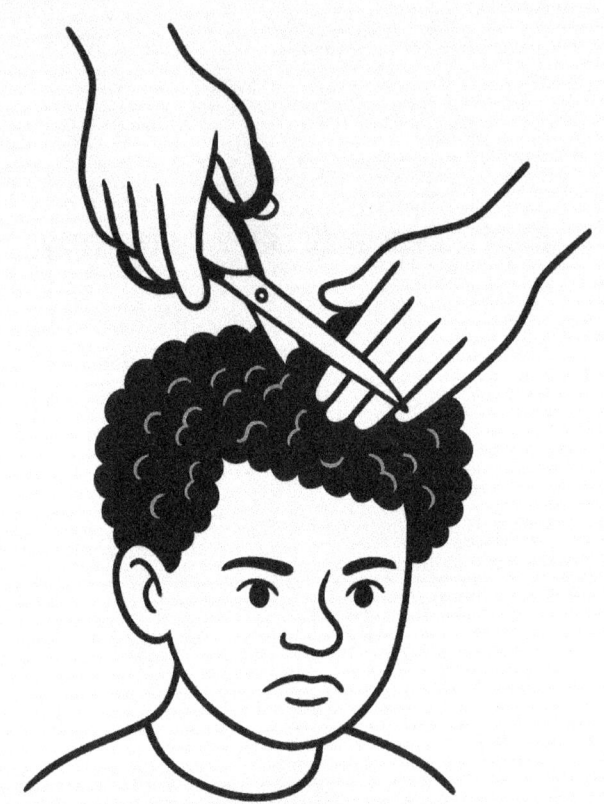

YOU CAN'T MOVE FORWARD WITHOUT A CLEAN CUT.

If you've ever spent time in a barbershop or salon, you know it's more than a place to get your hair done — it's therapy with clippers and combs. The cut or style might be the reason you came, but the conversations are the reason you stay.

In the chair, walls come down. You talk about everything — relationships, money, sports, politics, family drama, dreams you're chasing, fears you're carrying. Sometimes it's jokes flying back and forth. Other times, it gets deep, and before you realize it, you've said things you didn't even plan on sharing.

The magic of it is this: the barber or stylist isn't just fixing your hair — they're helping you carry your load. They listen. They laugh with you. They drop advice that hits harder than a motivational speaker. And the people sitting around? They chime in too, turning a simple appointment into a whole community session.

That's why these spaces matter. For a lot of us, the barbershop and salon are the only places we feel safe enough to be raw and real. They remind us that we don't have to deal with life alone. The cut heals the outside, but the conversation heals the inside.

"The chair ain't just for cuts — it's for conversations."

12

The Gender Hair Divide

From the time we're kids, hair comes with rules. Boys get told to keep it short and "clean." Girls get told to keep it neat, long, and "feminine." Step outside those boxes, and suddenly you're "doing too much" or "not looking right."

Maybe you were that boy who wanted twists or locs but kept hearing,

"That's not professional."

Or maybe you were that girl who wanted to cut it short but got told,

"Don't cut your hair, boys won't like it."

The message is the same — your style is being policed by gender expectations that never asked what you actually wanted.

The weight of those rules hits hard. For guys, hair becomes tied to masculinity, toughness, or respectability. For women, it becomes tied to beauty, worth, and desirability. But the truth is, hair doesn't belong to gender. Hair is just hair — expression, creativity, identity. The rules? Those were made up.

And when you finally step outside of those limits, there's freedom. A boy growing locs. A girl buzzing her head. A person rocking whatever style feels true to them. That's when hair stops being a cage and starts being a canvas.

Because at the end of the day, your hair doesn't care what box society tries to put it in. It only cares how you choose to wear it.

"Hair don't got a gender, people do."

13

Hair & Relationships

Hair has a funny way of showing up in relationships. Sometimes it's love — a partner running their hands through your curls, hyping you up after a fresh cut, or reminding you how good you look when you don't even see it yourself. Those little moments feel big, because they confirm what you hope is true: that you're attractive, seen, and accepted as you are.

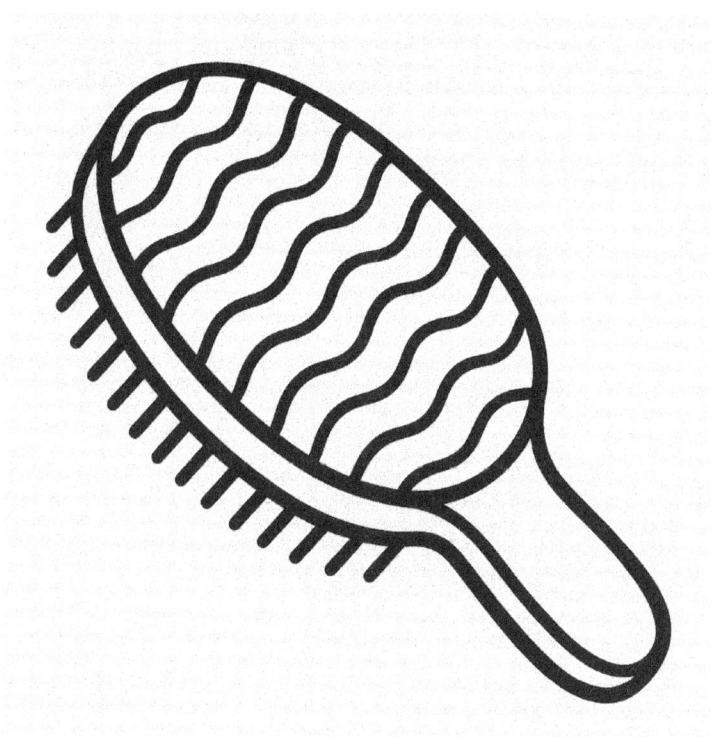

But sometimes, it cuts the other way. Maybe they joked about your hair being "too nappy." Maybe they suggested you wear it straighter, longer, shorter — anything but the way you wanted. And even if they didn't mean harm, it plants a seed of doubt. It makes you second-guess your style, your beauty, your worth.

The truth is, hair in relationships isn't just about looks — it's about respect. A partner who loves you should love your hair too, because your hair is part of you. Criticism disguised as "preference" isn't love. It's control. And control has no place in real connection.

When someone embraces you fully — twists, fades, wigs, locs, braids, natural — that's love. And when they don't? That's your reminder that the most important relationship is the one you have with yourself. Because when you accept your hair, no outside opinion can shake you.

"If they can't love your hair, they can't love you."

14

Hair & Aging

The first time you spot a gray hair, it catches you off guard. You lean closer to the mirror like,

"Wait... is that really there?"

Some people pluck it out fast. Others laugh it off. But deep down, it feels like more than just a strand — it feels like a reminder that time is moving.

For men, it might be that receding hairline or thinning at the crown. For women, it could be shedding or hair losing its thickness. No matter how it shows up, aging hair has a way of making us reflect on more than just appearance. It makes us think about who we were, who we are, and who we're becoming.

And that's what makes it tough. Because we live in a world obsessed with staying young. Dye it, cover it, fix it, hide it. The message is clear: aging is something to fight. But the truth is, aging isn't loss — it's evolution. Those grays are proof you've lived, learned, and survived. Those changes are markers of growth, not weakness.

It doesn't mean you can't dye, cut, or style your hair however you want. But it does mean you get to choose whether you see age as a flaw or as wisdom shining through. Hair may change with time, but confidence has no expiration date.

"Every gray is a stripe of wisdom."

15

Money, Hair & Hustle

Let's be real — keeping up with hair costs money. Wigs, bundles, braids, twists, weekly fades, products, edge control, oils, appointments — it all adds up quick. Some folks got a whole budget just for their hair, and even then, it feels like it's never enough.

We don't always say it out loud, but there's pressure behind those prices. You want to look fresh, because hair is confidence. You want to keep up with trends, because hair is status. But the grind of spending can leave you stressed, broke, or feeling like you're chasing an image you can't afford.

The truth is, hair has always been part of the hustle. Barbers, stylists, braiders — they've built whole businesses around it. And as customers, we sometimes sacrifice more than we should just to keep up appearances. But what happens when chasing a look starts draining your peace?

Here's the real flex: **Balance.** Taking care of yourself without letting it wreck your pockets. Loving your natural hair enough that you don't always need the "extras." Investing in your mental health as much as your maintenance. Because when the bills are paid and the stress is low, you glow differently.

Your worth has never been in the price tag of your style. The sharpest cut, the longest bundle, the freshest install — none of that can compete with real confidence.

"If it costs your peace, it's too expensive."

16

Hair as Celebration

Not every hair story is about struggle. Some of the best memories are tied to celebration. Think about it — prom nights, graduations, weddings, birthdays, holidays. Before the big moment, there's always the hair appointment. The braids getting done, the curls being set, the line-up sharp enough to slice the air.

In those moments, hair becomes part of the ritual. It's how we prepare ourselves for joy. Families gather around, laughing, sharing stories while someone's getting braided. Friends gas each other up before heading out. A fresh style isn't just about looking good — it's about marking the occasion.

And beyond the big events, there's everyday celebration too. That feeling of trying a new style and loving it. That confidence when you finally nail a routine that works. Or just the simple joy of walking outside and letting the sun hit your fresh cut or twist-out.

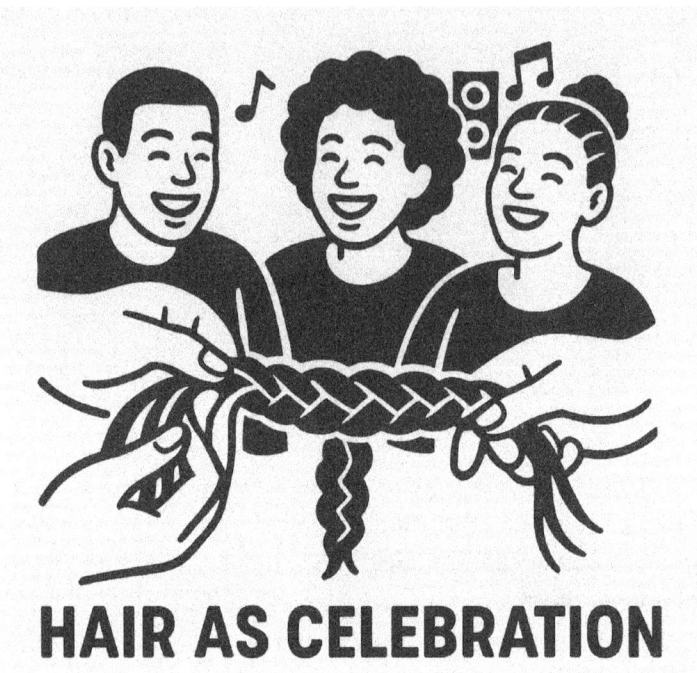

HAIR AS CELEBRATION

Hair has always been a way we show pride in ourselves and in our culture. Styles passed down through generations, creativity that never stops evolving, the boldness to wear it how we want. It's more than maintenance — it's art, it's memory, it's love.

So don't forget to celebrate your hair story, even in the small moments. Every style tells a story, and every story is worth honoring.

HAIR AS CELEBRATION

"Every style tells a story worth celebrating."

IV

Society, Culture & Connection

17

Myths We Grew Up On

Everybody grew up hearing wild things about hair.
  "Don't go outside with your hair wet, you'll get sick."
  "Brushing your hair a hundred times makes it grow."
  "Grease fixes everything."
  "If you cut it, it'll grow back faster."

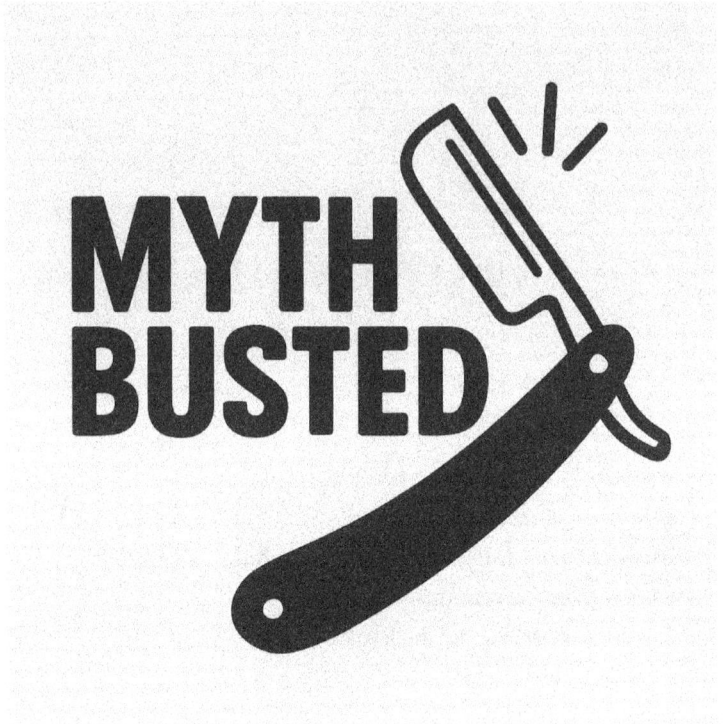

At the time, it all sounded official because it came from someone older — a parent, an auntie, a barber, a neighbor. But looking back, half of it was myth, passed down like family recipes nobody ever fact-checked. Some of it was harmless. Some of it? It actually did more harm than good.

Because here's the thing: myths don't just shape how we treat our hair — they shape how we think about it. They taught us to fear certain textures, to believe certain styles were "unruly," or to think some hair was automatically "better" than others. And those ideas stick longer than we realize.

Breaking myths isn't just about calling them out — it's about unlearning what doesn't serve us anymore. It's about replacing old beliefs with truth. And the truth is, no one way of wearing your hair is more valid than another. Healthier routines, self-acceptance, and confidence matter way more than old sayings.

So laugh at the funny ones, let go of the harmful ones, and keep what actually works for you. Just because it's been said for years doesn't mean it needs to be carried any further.

"Just 'cause grandma said it don't mean it's gospel."

18

Slay The Day, The Hair Way

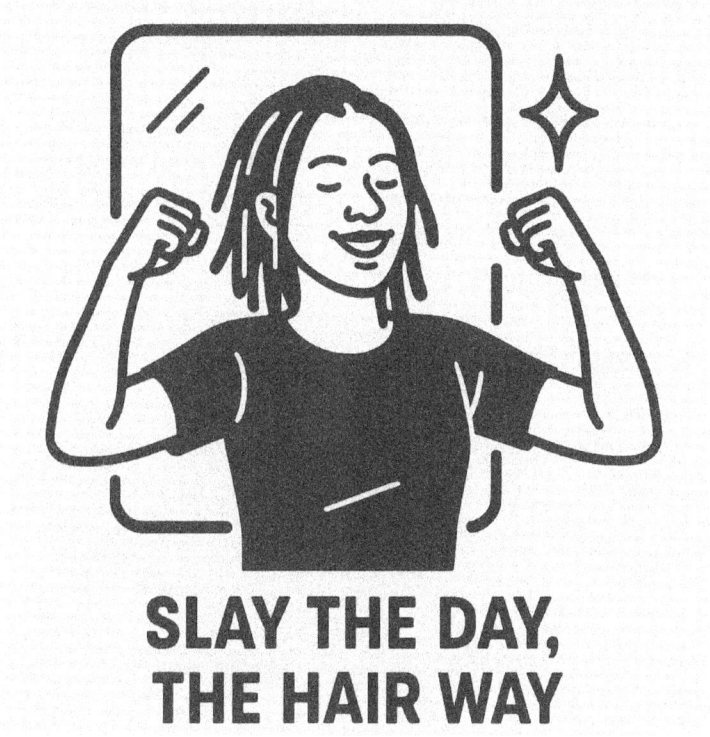

SLAY THE DAY, THE HAIR WAY

There's a shift that happens the moment you stop letting your hair define you and start letting it remind you. Instead of chasing every style to prove something, you wear what feels true to you. Instead of worrying about every comment, you walk out the door already knowing who you are.

That's the power of embracing your hair — not because it's perfect, but because it's yours. Locs, fades, wigs, braids, curls, silk presses — none of it matters more than the confidence you carry with it. Hair can't create your worth. It can only highlight the worth that's already there.

When you realize that, the game changes. You stop apologizing for how you show up. You stop comparing your journey to someone else's. And suddenly, the same mirror that once felt like a critic becomes your biggest hype man.

Because slaying the day isn't about a flawless twist-out or a fresh taper. It's about walking into the world knowing you belong in every room you step into. The style just adds flavor to the confidence you already built.

So whatever your look is today — rock it. Own it. Live it. The world doesn't need another version of somebody else. It needs the version of you that only you can bring.

"Confidence is the best product you'll ever wear."

Epilogue

By now, you've probably realized this was never just about hair. Every story, every lesson, every laugh and heavy moment was really about something deeper — how we see ourselves, how we carry our confidence, and how we take care of our minds.

Hair was just the mirror. The real reflection has always been you.

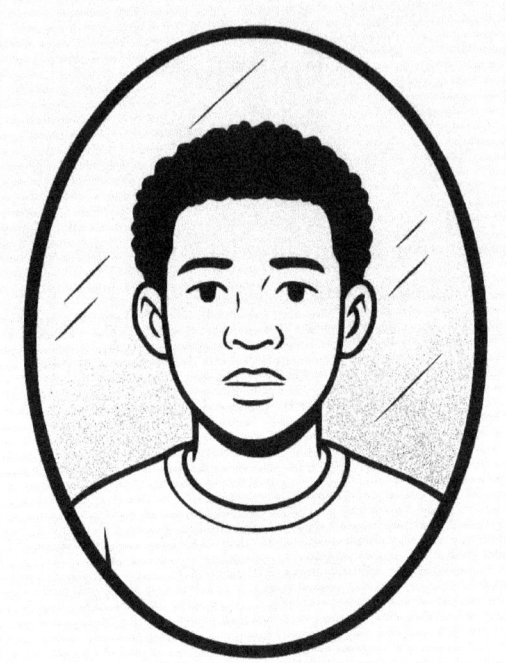

At the end of the day, it's not about the hair – it's about the head it's on.

So when you step back into your own life — into the barbershop chair, into the salon, into the bathroom mirror on a random Tuesday morning — remember what these pages showed you. The bad cuts, the big chops, the slow growth, the celebrations, the myths, the pressure, the freedom. They're all part of the journey.

Your hair will change a hundred times over the years. Styles will come and go. Trends will fade. But the one thing that never goes out of style is self-acceptance. When you carry that, every look you rock is powerful, because it's backed by something real.

So here's the takeaway: love your hair, but love yourself more. Because no matter what's on your head, what really matters is the head it's on.

"At the end of the day, it's not about the hair — it's about the head it's on."

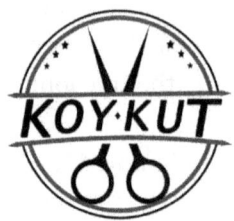

About the Author

Koy Kut is a master barber, storyteller, and creative who knows that a haircut is never just a haircut — it's confidence, culture, and conversation. After years behind the chair listening to stories, sharing laughs, and watching the way people light up after a fresh style, he realized hair and mental health are more connected than most people think.

Through his books and work, Koy Kut uses everyday experiences — from barbershop therapy to the natural hair journey — to spark deeper conversations about identity, confidence, and self-love. His mission is simple: to remind people that hair grows, styles change, but how you carry yourself lasts forever.

www.ingramcontent.com/pod-product-compliance
Lightning Source LLC
Chambersburg PA
CBHW050918160426
43194CB00011B/2452